HOW TO COPE WITH DISTRESSING VOICES

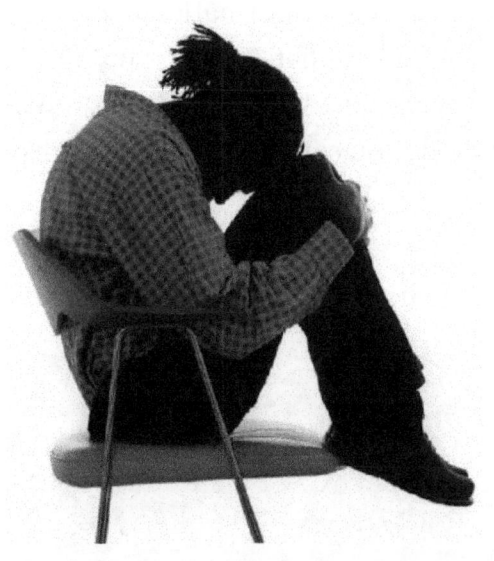

By Patricia A Carlisle

Introduction

I want to thank you and congratulate you for choosing the book, *"How to Cope with Distressing Voices"*.

This book contains proven steps and strategies on how to deal with the voices in your head. It has everything you need to know about hearing voices.

This book contains useful information about voices or auditory hallucinations, and what their possible causes and complications are. This book also talks about the various treatment methods you can use to cope with distressing voices.

Thanks again for choosing this book, I hope you enjoy it!

ABOUT THE AUTHOR
PATRICIA A. CARLISLE, MSW, CBT

Patricia Carlisle- a Master Social Worker and Cognitive Behavioral Therapist (CBT) gives out an expression of how important it is for an individual to take into consideration the concept of self-assessment to know what human, technical and conceptual skills they posses to perform or to achieve what they desire, or to deal with everyday life. However, every particular group of people has their own unique set of ideas, traditions and events including the frame of mind according to which people perform but there are many who faces problems and fail to maintain a healthy mind set affecting their behaviors and performance to those around them.

People like Patricia Carlisle are among those who have felt this urge of serving people and helping them out of their mental crisis towards a healthy life. She has experienced some close encounters in her personal life regarding mental health issues in her family and friends that has encouraged her to pursue this as her career.

Currently Patricia Carlisle is serving as a Certified On-Line Cognitive Behavioral Therapist with an extensive 15years of experience using Cognitive-Behavior Therapy Techniques. She envisions a world where everyone gets mental health treatment with no mental health stigma and to make it real she has already set up her own Holistic Measure Online Comprehensive Behavioral Healthcare Company after retiring from The Nord Center in The Partial Hospitalization Program (PHP) Dept for 5 years and Murtis H. Taylor Mental Health Center as a mental health counselor, psychological support technician and case manager for 10 years to emulsify her skills more professionally.

Along with this, she has wrote down her passion as a clinician in 25 or more short books to help individuals and families get their life back, freeing them of the restraints of negative thinking, anxiety and depression by using different approaches. She is highly appreciated among her clients for her flexibility and professionalism of dealing with them graciously. To reach her, make use of her direct website address: http://therapist2013.wix.com/e-therapy . As she is ready to inspire hope and contribute to health and well-being by providing the best online health care through comprehensive practice, education and research.

TABLE OF CONTENT

Chapter 1:

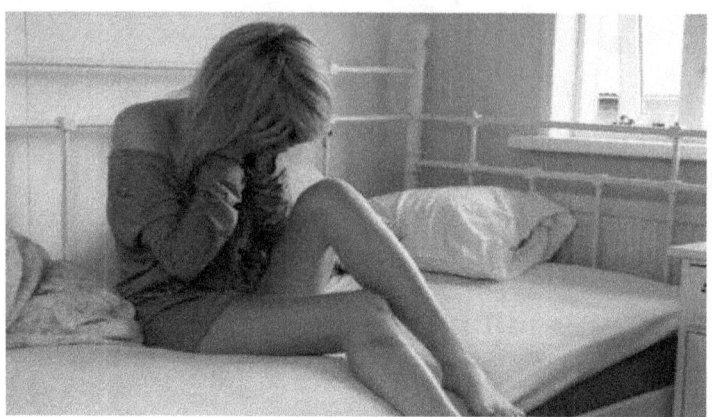

HEARING VOICES

Hearing voices is relatively common. According to statistics, between three and ten percent of people in the United States hear voices at a point in their lives. So when you hear voices, do not immediately freak out because it does not mean that you have a mental illness. If you are struggling with coping with these voices, you may need support or help.

How does it feel to Hear Voices?

It can be difficult to describe what it is like to hear distressing voices. It may be there all day, preventing you from doing even the simplest chores. If the voices get worse, they may stress you out if you do not follow what they say. Worse, they may tell you to hurt, or kill yourself or other people. This is why some people blame the voices in their heads when they do something terrible. Some of the more famous ones include Joan of Arc, Socrates, Mahatma Ghandi, Carl Jung, and Anthony Hopkins.

Hearing voices in your head may be the same as hearing the voices of other people through your ears, except that there is no physical source. Nonetheless, just like normal voices, every experience is different. For instance, you may leave a party, or isolate yourself from other people because the voices tell you to. You may also think that someone is calling your name even when no one else is around you.

According to researchers, those who are in mourning are most susceptible to hearing voices in their head. They think that they hear the voices of their deceased loved ones. Also, just like hearing voices through your ears, you may also hear voices as if they are thoughts that enter your mind. Do not misinterpret this as an idea that comes from your own mind. Such voices typically come from thoughts that are not your own.

For instance, you may recall a tune or rhyme, and repeat it under your breath unconsciously, causing it to repeat in your head over and over. You may even catch yourself humming or whistling to it. You did not really think about it, and yet it is hard to get it out of your head.

The difference between "voice thoughts", and tunes is that the former may coherently speak to you, and encourage you to participate in the conversation. Since you did not think of it, you do not know what it is going to tell you.

You can hear these voices in various ways. You can experience them inside your head, in your body, or from outside your head. There can be many different voices, or just one. They may talk about you or talk to you directly. These voices are just like dreams.

When you are bored, you can drift away and have a dream. In your dream, anything can happen to you, and you may believe that they are real. This is just like hearing voices. It is like you are having a dream while you are awake.

Hearing Voices Then and Now

Voices or auditory hallucinations were once believed to be heard only by people with schizophrenia. People back then also thought that such voices cannot be understood, and do not make any sense, and that people who hear voices need to take medication. They also thought that talking about the experience can lead to worse consequences.

Engaging in the voices was discouraged on the notion that doing so will contribute to the hearer's delusions. Those who heard voices, and did not respond well to medication were isolated.

Today, experts prove that anyone can hear these voices, not just those with schizophrenia. Dr. Patricia Deegan, an expert in clinical psychology, said that she has heard voices for a long time. Because of this, she developed, Developing Empathy for the Lived Experience of Psychiatric Disability: A Simulation of Hearing Distressing Voices, which is a three-hour workshop and groundbreaking training that enables mental health professionals to understand deeply the challenges that people who hear distressing voices face.

During the workshop, the participants listen to a lecture about hearing voices recorded by Dr. Deegan. Then, they listen to an audiotape of distressing voices through their headphones. While listening, they complete a series of mock tasks of activities, such as cognitive testing, psychiatric emergency room interview, day treatment activities, and social interaction within a community.

Afterwards, the participants have a dramatic experience of what it is like to hear distressing voices. Dr. Jim Willow, a psychiatric resident at the PsycHealth Centre in Winnipeg, said that after participating in the workshop, he realized that he had been treating schizophrenia for years, yet he never really known about it. He added that he did not have true empathy, or wisdom until he attended the workshop.

The learning objectives of the workshop are to learn about the varieties and types of voice-hearing experiences; to know more ways on how to help individuals who hear distressing voices; and to have more understanding and empathy regarding the voice-hearing experiences.

Additional Research on Hearing Voices

A lot of people who hear voices have never had a mental illness. In fact, a huge number of the population hears occasional and brief voices during times of bereavement, separation, and divorce. Those who are in extreme circumstances also tend to hear voices. Eighty percent of people who have suffered torture as well as long-distance yachtsmen experience hallucinations.

According to an epidemiological research done in Baltimore, ten to fifteen percent of fifteen thousand participants said that they have heard voices, but only one-third of them experienced negative effects. In addition, a research conducted in 1991 have found that many of the cases regarding hearing distressing voices were not able to meet the criteria for psychiatric diagnosis.

A research done by Dr. Marius Romme, has also showed that both patients and non-patients who hear voices hear positive and negative voices at a similar level. However, the patients tend to be more upset, and more afraid of the voices than the non-patients.

The Aspects of Voices

In general, there are five aspects of voices: situation, thoughts and images, body or physical sensations, moods or emotions, and behaviors. It is important for you to know the answer to the following questions:

Situation

- When did you hear the voices?
- Where were you when you heard the voices?
- Who were you with when you heard the voices?
- What happened when you heard the voices?
- Were the voices loud?
- How many voices are there?
- How powerful were the voices?
- What did the voices tell you?
- Did you experience other hallucinations, involving your sense of sight, touch, or smell, when you heard the voices?
- How frequent did the voices talk to you?

Thoughts and Images

- What immediately went through your mind when the voices said what they said?
- Did you agree with what the voices said?
- If you agreed, what did the voices say or mean about you?
- What is the worst thing about what the voices said?
- How can you explain what they said?
- What is their purpose for telling you that?

- How did you make sense of what the voices said?

Body or Physical Sensations

- What did you feel when you heard the voices?
- Where did you feel it?
- Was there anything else you noticed with your body when you heard the voices?

Moods or Emotions

- What emotions did you have when you heard the voices?
- How intense were your feelings?

Behaviors

- What did you do when you heard the voices?
- What did you not do when you heard the voices?
- What were your automatic reactions when you heard the voices?
- What did you feel like doing when you heard the voices?
- What did other people see you doing when you heard the voices?
- What helped you cope and get through the experience?

Causes of Hearing Voices

Hearing voices may be associated with certain medical conditions and psychiatric disorders. It may also be associated with substance abuse and withdrawal, sensory loss, medications, severe fatigue, and lack of sleep.

Certain psychiatric conditions, such as bipolar disorder, schizophrenia, schizoid personality disorder, psychotic depression, and schizotypal personality disorder, may also cause you to hear voices.

Other possible causes include delirium, brain tumor, dementia, seizure disorders, and hearing loss. In some cases, it may be a symptom of a life-threatening condition that must be evaluated immediately. Such life-threatening conditions include stroke, seizure, acute delirium, and severe infection.

Possible Complications of Hearing Voices

Since a serious illness may cause hearing voices, failure to receive medical treatment can result to permanent damage and serious complications. After diagnosing the underlying cause, it is crucial to follow the treatment plan in order to reduce the risk of certain complications. These complications include coma, brain damage, drug overdose, alcohol poisoning, drug abuse, alcohol abuse, self-harm, increase risk of injury, violence, suicide, financial or legal problems, and difficulties at school, work, and with relationships.

Chapter 2:

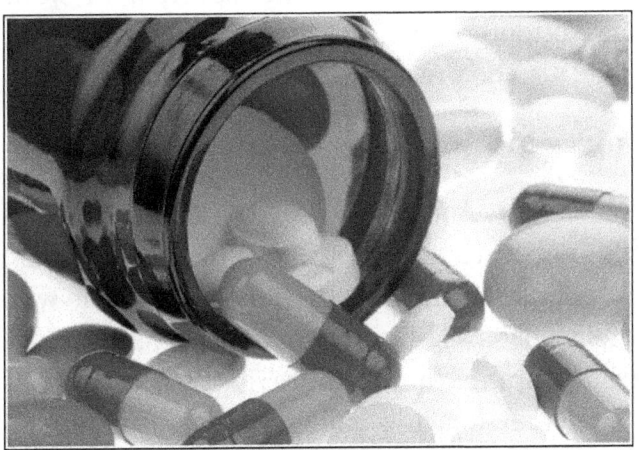

MEDICATIONS AND SUPPORT

If you are hearing voices and are thinking of seeing a doctor, ask yourself these questions:

- Do you feel desperate and can no longer carry on?

- Do you hurt yourself or lash out at other people because of the voices in your head?

- Are you confused or struggling to focus due to your experiences?

- Are you scared or frightened because of such experiences?

- Do you struggle to study or work because of the voices in your head?

If you answer 'yes' to any of these questions, you have to talk to someone about your feelings. You may see a general practitioner, or go to a specialist. General practitioners generally refer patients to mental health professionals. The services you need may depend on the severity of your condition. You may undergo cognitive behavioral therapy, or counseling. You may also be prescribed with medication.

The Hearing Voices Movement

The Hearing Voices Movement refers to individuals, and organizations that advocate the Hearing Voices Approach, which is a way of understanding the experiences of people who hear voices in their heads. The movement was founded by Patsy Hage, Marius Romme, and Sandra Escher in 1987. It challenges the belief that hearing voices is a sign of mental illness.

The Hearing Voices Movement regards hearing voices as an unusual yet understandable and meaningful human variation. Because of this, it rejects the pathologisation and stigma of hearing voices. Instead, it advocates social justice, support, and human rights for those who hear voices. It also challenges the legitimacy of the schizophrenia construct.

More and more psychiatrists are becoming open to the use of the Hearing Voices Approach, as well as willing to help individuals who hear voices understand their experience better with or without the involvement of medications.

For instance, the Critical Psychiatry Network, which is a network of medical students and psychiatrists, is sympathetic to the Hearing Voices Networks (HVN). The Hearing Voices Networks are peer-focused organizations for individuals who hear voices, or auditory hallucinations, and mental health professionals, activists, and family members who support them.

Do You Have to Take Medication?

It is up to you if you want to take medication or not. Some people find medications helpful in suppressing or lessening the distressing voices in their heads, while others do not see any improvement. Some also experience negative side effects when they take medications.

Before taking any medication, remind yourself that taking it will not fix the underlying problem. You have to realize that there are issues that tend to trigger such voices. Nonetheless, medications may work for you for either the short-term or the long term.

Antipsychotics

Antipsychotics are medications used for mental disorders. They can help with severe depression, extreme mood swings, thought disorder, delusions, and hearing voices. They affect the neurotransmitters or brain chemicals, particularly dopamine. These brain chemicals are responsible for making you feel satisfied, motivated, and significant. They are also involved in controlling the muscles.

Older antipsychotics, also referred to as first-generation antipsychotics, and typical antipsychotics, block the action of dopamine. If you take them, you may experience side effects, such as stiffness, shakiness, uncomfortable restlessness, breast swelling or tenderness, and dizziness.

Newer antipsychotics have only been in existence for over ten years. They also block dopamine, but not as strongly as older antipsychotics. They also affect the serotonin levels in the brain. These antipsychotics are also referred to as second-generation antipsychotics, and atypical antipsychotics.

If you take them, you may experience side effects such as weight gain, slowness, sleepiness, increased risk of diabetes, and dizziness. However, in comparison to the older antipsychotics, they are less likely to result to tardive dyskinesia, Parkinsonian side effects, and sexual dysfunction.

Who should you talk to?

It is a good idea to speak with someone you trust regarding the voices that you hear. You can confide to a friend, a family member, a spiritual leader, a counselor, or your partner. In the United Kingdom, hearing voices is often stigmatized. Because of this, most of the people who hear such voices feel that they have to keep their experience confidential.

Although perfectly understandable, it can still be difficult to keep a secret like this for a long time. What's more, it can be difficult to go about your life being afraid, or ashamed to tell other people about your experience.

Hence, you have to talk to someone who can understand what you are going through. If you are still hesitant to open up, you can chat with other people online. Find individuals who also experience the same thing. Talking to someone who knows exactly how it feels to hear voices is good for you.

Where Else can you Get Support

If you need support, you can contact help lines, peer support groups, and spiritual support groups. Do not try to keep things to yourself. Remember that there are people who are always willing to listen. If you feel embarrassed to speak face-to-face, you can dial a helpline.

You can also join online forums and message boards to interact with people from different parts of the world who understand your condition. Joining online communities is helpful since you can interact with other people who know exactly what you are going through.

There are no judgments, and you are free to share your experiences. Likewise, they can share their experiences with you, as well as give you information regarding studies and publications about auditory hallucinations.

You can also attend therapy or counseling. Seeing a therapist is ideal because this will let you receive customized treatment. You can receive individual or group therapy. Young people under eighteen years of age can avail of Child and Adolescent Mental Health Services (CAMHS), and Youth Counseling Services.

Chapter 3:

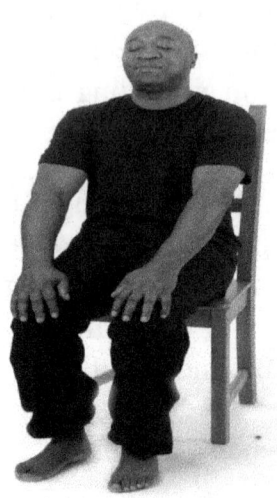

TECHNIQUES FOR COPING

To help you cope with distressing voices, you can try the following techniques. They are practically self-help techniques that you can do on your own, without the assistance of a medical professional. Some techniques may involve the help of a therapist or doctor.

Focusing Techniques

- You have to accept that the voices are not your problem, but rather they are the consequences of your real problem. To deal with this, you need to find out what makes you hear such voices.
- Be sure to identify these distressing voices. How many voices are there? Can you tell or assume the age and gender of the one talking to you? Find out as much as you can about these voices.

- You must also know which boundaries you can apply to the voices in your head. For instance, you may tell them to be quiet for now, and you will listen to them later.
- Do not just focus on the negative voices though. You must also listen to the positive ones.
- Set a specific time for listening to the voices in your head. This way, you can complete your chores without getting distracted.
- Tell the distressing voices that you will only answer them when they stop being disrespectful towards you.
- Allow someone you trust, such as your partner, friend, relative, or therapist, to directly speak with the voices.
- Write down the things that the voices tell you.

Positive Emotional Techniques

- Listen to invigorating music.
- Go out on a picnic.
- Review the list of things that you were able to accomplish.
- Look at photos in your photo albums.
- Create a list of your positive attributes according to other people.
- Create a list of your strengths and assets in your opinion.
- Stack up some candies in your drawer.
- Write letters or poems.
- Read good books.
- Motivate yourself with positive statements.
- Watch movies that make you feel good.

Emotional Focusing

- Talk to someone about your feelings.

- List down emotional triggers.
- Draw or paint your emotions.
- Write in your diary.
- Upload emotional poems on your blog.

Relaxation Techniques

- Acknowledge your fear, stress, or worry, and then let go of it.
- Count your breaths.
- Focus on your breathing.
- Take a walk outdoors.
- Dance.
- Practice guided visualization.
- Practice yoga.
- Go for a swim.
- Get a body massage.

Comforting Techniques

- Pick or buy some flowers.
- Change your bed sheets.
- Hug a teddy bear.
- Hug a person close to you.
- Eat your favorite food.
- Have a refreshing smoothie.
- Take a bubble bath.
- Squeeze a stress ball.
- Say a prayer.
- Sing a song.
- Play a musical instrument.
- Spray on some perfume.
- Inhale an essential oil.

Distraction Techniques

- Clean your room.
- Organize your closet.
- Exercise.
- Do some gardening.
- Play games on your computer.
- Hum a tune.
- Knit a sweater or mitten.
- Participate in sports.
- Call a friend.
- Visit a friend.
- Shop for new clothes, shoes, bags, etc.
- Walk in shallow water.

Additional Coping Mechanisms

- Chanting
- Acupuncture
- Sleeping
- Sex
- Meditation

Chapter 4:

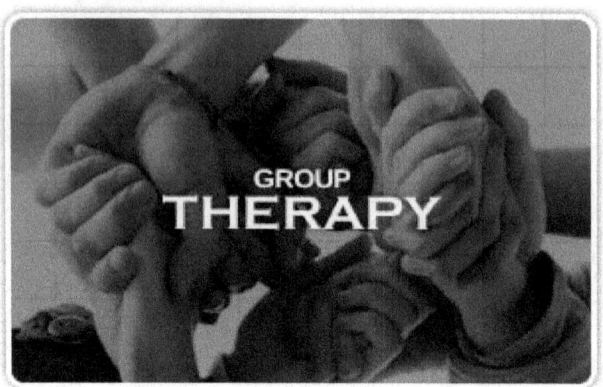

CBT, rTMS, and Enhanced Supportive Therapy for Distressing Voices

Talking therapies, such as Cognitive Behavioral Therapy (CBT), can help you cope with distressing voices. Cognitive behavioral therapy has been found to be effective in reducing the level of distress, and frequency of auditory hallucinations, especially when there are other psychotic symptoms present.

Enhanced Supportive Therapy has also been found to reduce the frequency of such auditory hallucinations as well as the violent resistance that patients display towards the voices in their heads. This treatment method has also been found to cause an overall decrease in the malignancy of these hallucinations.

Although not recommended by the National Institute for Health and Care Excellence (NICE), the Repetitive Transcranial Magnetic Stimulation (rTMS) has been found to be helpful in reducing distressing voices. It involves the use of an electromagnet that sends out magnetic pulses on the scalp. Such pulses pass through the skull to stimulate a portion of the brain. The activity in this portion of the brain is reduced by low frequency transcranial magnetic stimulation. Do not worry because the procedure is painless. You will remain conscious during the duration of the procedure.

Cognitive Behavioral Therapy

For people who hear distressing voices, cognitive behavioral therapy may be ideal. In fact, the NICE recommends it along with antipsychotic drugs. You will notice more improvement in your condition if you combine cognitive behavioral therapy with medication.

Again, you have to realize that cognitive behavioral therapy cannot get rid of your problems. Nevertheless, it can help you deal with the voices better, since it is based on the concept that your feelings, thoughts, actions, and physical sensations are all interrelated, and that your negative feelings and thoughts can keep you trapped in a vicious cycle.

When you undergo cognitive behavioral therapy, you will be put through assessment. You will be asked to express your thoughts about your experiences. Your therapist will use scales to rate and monitor your progress. If your life is somewhat chaotic, you can greatly benefit from written materials and diagrams.

After assessment comes the engagement stage. Your therapist will tell you what the session is about. Throughout the session, you will undergo Socratic questioning to help you understand your situation, and find out how you can cope with it through guided discovery.

Your therapist will use a vulnerability-stress model to help you know that vulnerability is a vigorous concept that is affected by different factors, such as physical illnesses, and life events.

Your therapist will also tell you that he cannot give you answers, but he can explain things to you if you cooperate.

The ABC model was developed by Ellis and Harper. It helps patients organize their confusing experiences. It involves a series of steps that will help the patients clarify the connections between their emotional distress and beliefs.

Repetitive Transcranial Magnetic Stimulation

Ralph Hoffman and his colleagues from the Department of Psychiatry in Yale conducted a study about the effects of low frequency repetitive transcranial magnetic stimulation on auditory hallucinations. Note that repetitive transcranial magnetic stimulation is a non-invasive brain stimulation technique.

It is not the same as electroconvulsive therapy (ECT). You will not feel any discomfort when you undergo the procedure. You will simply experience a tapping sensation on your scalp. As for the side effects, do not worry because they are minimal. You may only experience some minor facial twitching, and headaches.

Repetitive transcranial magnetic stimulation makes use of a magnetic field to induce electric currents in the cortex. In the study, the left tempoproparietal cortex was targeted because it is the area responsible for language and voice hearing.

Conclusion

Thank you again for choosing this book!

I hope this book was able to help you learn ways on how to cope with the voices in your head.

The next step is to apply what you have learned from this book.

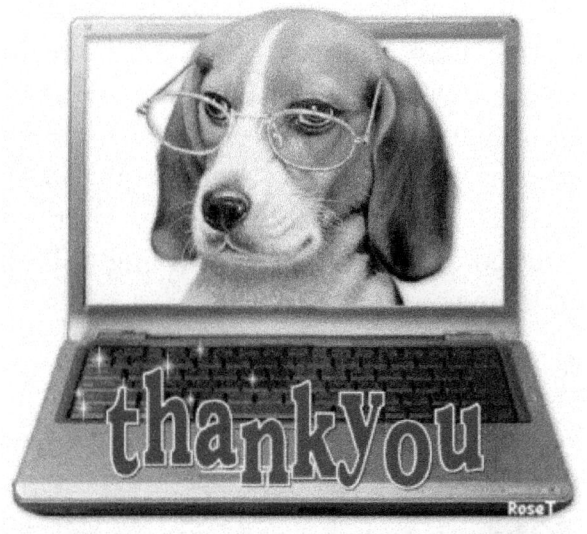

Finally, if you enjoyed this book would you be kind enough to leave a review for this book on Amazon? It'd be greatly appreciated!

Thank you and good luck!

Preview Of 'Stress Solutions: Proven methods on how to live without worry'

Chapter 1
WRITE YOUR WORRIES DOWN

Writing down all of your anxiety and problems before an important exam may facilitate decreasing of test-taking worry, in line with a 2011 study in Science. Although exams aren't any longer a serious problem to most of the people, an associate professor in psychology at the University of Chicago stated that this approach may work for individuals facing anxieties about different things. Moreover writing down your worries allow you to let go the burden of keeping track of your problems in your mind. It will be easier to just write down and review and think about the solutions for your worries in a designated period of time rather than trying to keep record of all your worries in your mind.

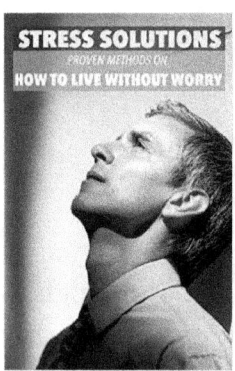

check out the rest of (Stress Solutions: Proven methods on how to live without worry) on Amazon.com

Check Out My Other Books

Below you'll find some of my other popular books that are popular on Amazon and Kindle as well. Alternatively, you can visit my author page on Amazon to see other work done by me.

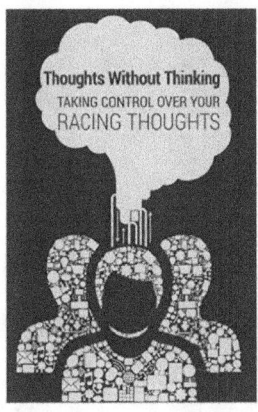

Thoughts Without Thinking: Taking control over your racing thoughts.

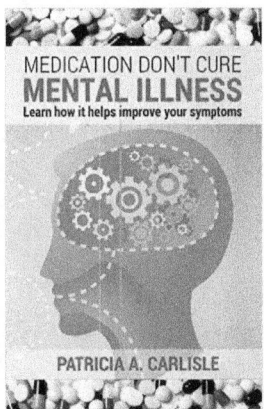

MEDICATION DON'T CURE MENTAL ILLNESS: Learn how it helps improve your symptoms.

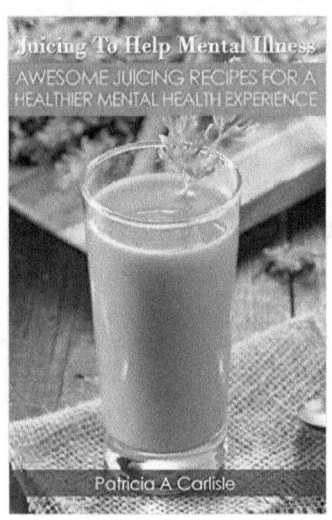

Juicing to help mental illness: Awesome juicing recipes for a healthier mental health.

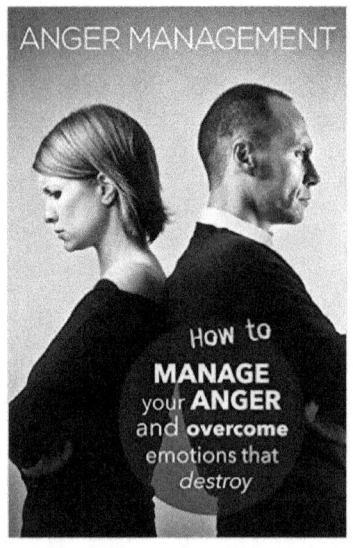

Anger Management: How to manage your anger and overcome emotions that destroy.

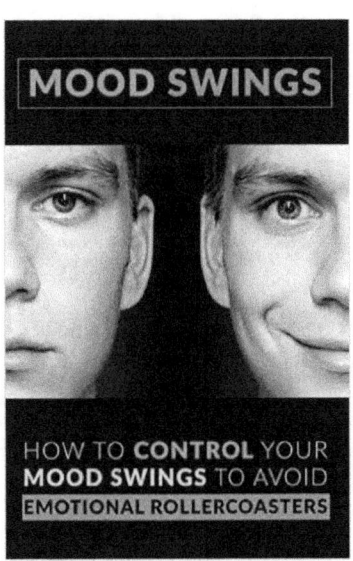

Mood Swings: How to control your mood swings to avoid emotional rollercoster's.

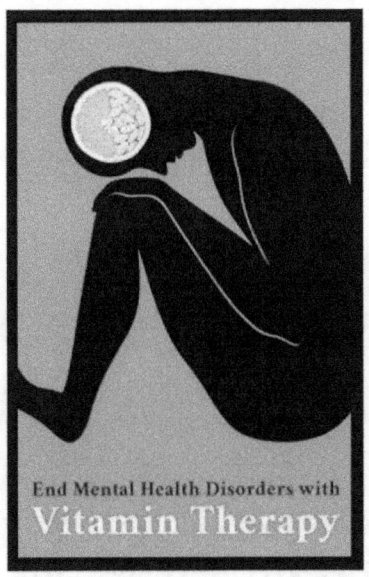

End Mental Disorders with vitamin therapy

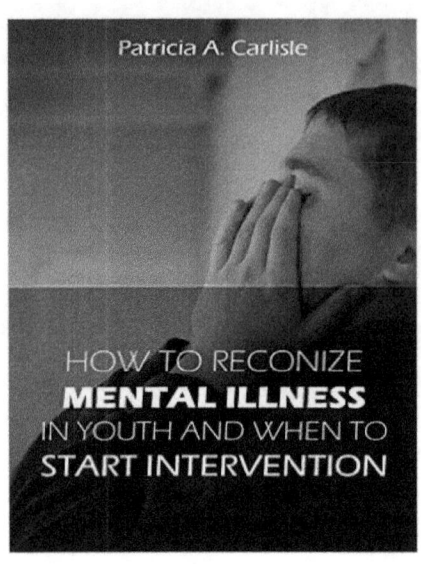

HOW TO RECOGNIZE MENTAL ILLNESS IN YOUTH AND WHEN TO START INTERVENTION.

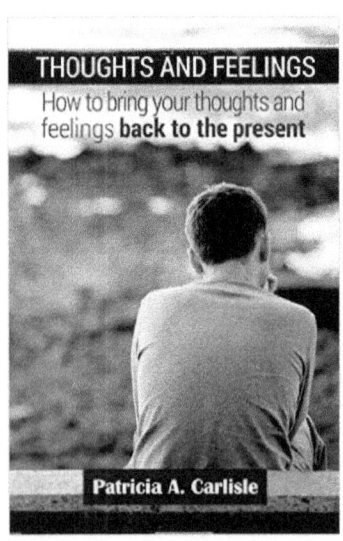

THOUGHTS AND FEELINGS: HOW TO BRING YOUR THOUGHTS AND FEELINGS BACK TO THE PRESENT.

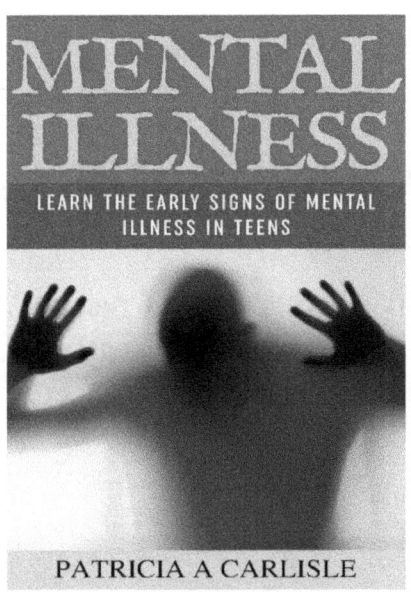

MENTAL ILLNESS: LEARN THE EARLY SIGNS OF MENTAL ILLNESS IN TEENS.

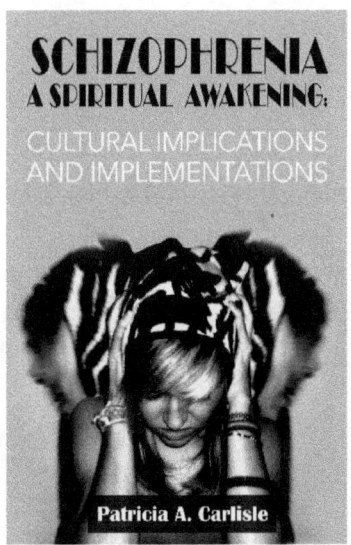

SCHIZOPHRENIA A SPIRITUAL AWAKENING: CULTURAL IMPLICATIONS AND IMPLEMENTATIONS

BONUS: SUBSCRIBE TO THE FREE BOOK

Beginners Guide to Yoga & Meditation

"Stressed out? Do You Feel Like The World Is Crashing Down Around You? Want To Take A Vacation That Will Relax Your Mind, Body And Spirit? Well this Easy To Read Step By Step

E-Book Makes It All Possible!"

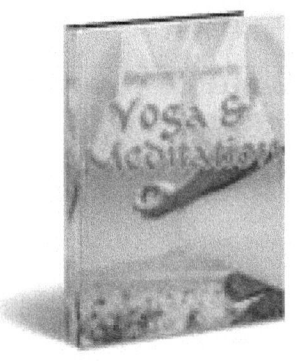

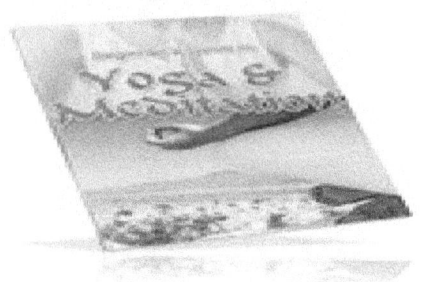

Instructions on how to join our mailing list, and receive a free copy of "Yoga and Meditation" can be found in any of my Kindle eBooks.

NOTE

NOTE

NOTE

NOTES

NOTES

NOTES